"Meditation is a gentle force of nature which brings contentment to the unruly mind"

Baba Ananda

Dedicated to Esme Hawk Ladygo

And Avery Jai Hayward

Produced by Hayward's Yoga in State College

220A S. Allen Street State College, PA. 16801

 ISBN 9780972111621

CONTENTS

Introduction

The object of meditation is to stop the mind from wandering all over the place and to sustain a single pointed focus for an extended period of time. This experience begins with concentration and then moves to another level which is recognizable and beneficial.

I challenge you to think of one color. Next, without fail, mentally repeat that color name, feel that color, or mentally picture that color for 60 seconds without intermission. Do it without the mind straying to any other thought whatsoever. At the same time feel the coolness of your inhalation thru the nose and hear the escape of your exhalation thru the mouth.

The list of instructions could continue until you were totally absorbed in all of your mental, physical and spiritual capacities all at once.

If you were able to keep that single pointed focus on that one color for 3 minutes, then the instructions in this book will seem very elementary. If; however, your mind started to wander after about 15 or 20 seconds then the instructions in this book will be of great benefit. Later, in this book, you will see a time line of a typical meditation experience.

Three minutes pass by very quickly. The older we get the quicker 3 minutes seem to pass.

The challenge given in this book is to experience meditation for a full three minutes without intermission.

Meditation is the single pointed focus that resides within the stillness of the mind. To experience meditation for three minutes may be difficult; but, as a goal, it is completely within our grasp.

Many questions crop up about meditation and the answers often evade us or are hidden deep in lengthy books or concealed from common view just enough to keep us from becoming aware of how to recognize the experience of meditation.

Many of us want to meditate but we don't know how. It is also possible that we are meditating but yet don't know it.

This compact book was written to help those who wish to achieve a state of meditation and to recognize that we have indeed already experienced meditation.

The instruction being delivered here comes from 10 years of Yoga practice and teaching in what is known as "Happy Valley", home of Penn State University, nestled between the mountains of Central Pennsylvania. A lot of the tips in this book are borrowed from the observation and teachings of others. I do not claim all the ideas in this book as my own and

wish to offer credit to those who have come before me offering insight into the experience of meditation. On the other hand, many of the tips given here are being written about as a result of my own first hand experiences and for those experiences I am indeed grateful.

Almost everyone has the ability to meditate. Meditation is easier for some than for others; however, once we gain a clear understanding of what meditation is, what it feels like before, during and after, then perhaps many of the clouds are lifted and meditation can be experienced more frequently and to greater benefit.

Meditation can be experienced while standing, sitting, or lying down. It can be experienced while our body is in motion or while the body is still. We can meditate while there are other sounds around us; traffic, music, conversation, birds, drums and laughter. In short, we meditate while the ears are still picking up sounds. We can meditate while we are feeling wind, coolness, heat, dryness, humidity, the sun and the rain. Actually we meditate while the sense of touch is picking up feeling. We can meditate while the eyes are opened or closed. We can meditate while looking at the sky, the grass, the clouds or a candle. We can meditate while looking out the

window or into complete darkness, or the darkness that we experience when we close our eyes. Indeed we meditate while the sense of sight is still picking up images. The ability of our mind to come to a single focus is what distinguishes meditation from other active mental states.

We can meditate while we taste something sweet or sour. We can meditate when our palate is moist or some what dry. We mediate while our taste buds are still detecting some flavor. We can meditate while we smell flowers, mustiness, incense or other aromas. In short we can meditate while the sense of smell is still

detecting something either on our around ourselves.

We can meditate while we are mentally engaged in problems and emotions, whether we are happy or sad. By nature we meditate while the mind is still active.

Meditation occurs while all the senses are fully operational and the mind is active. As you read further you will understand how.

Meditation has a timeline and it can be understood with the following examples and drawings.

Take three minutes at some point during the day that you decide you would like to meditate. Say for example that the first two minutes of meditation we have the eyes open, are looking around at our belongings or at nature. All kinds of thoughts and sensations are occurring that we are aware of, and seem to offer a distraction to our intended purpose. Then, for a few moments, our mind stops filtering our sensual input and our conscious thoughts become a little less active. All of a sudden an impulse from one of our senses, a thought, or an emotion attracts the conscious mind and it becomes active again. Three minutes or so has passed and yet we feel as if we have not meditated and we have lost control of our mission. Perhaps another few minutes pass with lots of mental activity and other sensual

impulses occurring and then there is a period where all this slows down again and we sense some stillness for a moment or two.

The Train

Here is an analogy: We are outdoors near a railroad track and a train approaches. We hear it coming, getting louder and louder; we can feel the rumble, see the approaching engine, smell the diesel fumes, and perhaps taste the exhaust. Now the train is right in front of us, traveling at a decent speed. As the train passes us we become totally absorbed in train. Everything is train. TRAIN, TRAIN, TRAIN. Nothing can distract us because the train is capturing our total attention and although we are safe, it is so close, right in front of us. Gradually, the train passes us completely and all the sights, sounds and feelings begin to

dissipate and fade away. In a few moments we can't hear it anymore, see it anymore, or feel it anymore. For a few moments, everything is still; even the thoughts of the passing train go away. And then we begin to perceive another train coming just a few miles away and the whole process starts again.

The reason I gave this analogy is that during the train episode there were a few moments when we were meditating. One when we were totally absorbed in TRAIN, TRAIN, TRAIN and again in the gap between the trains, when there was stillness, right before the perception of the next train.

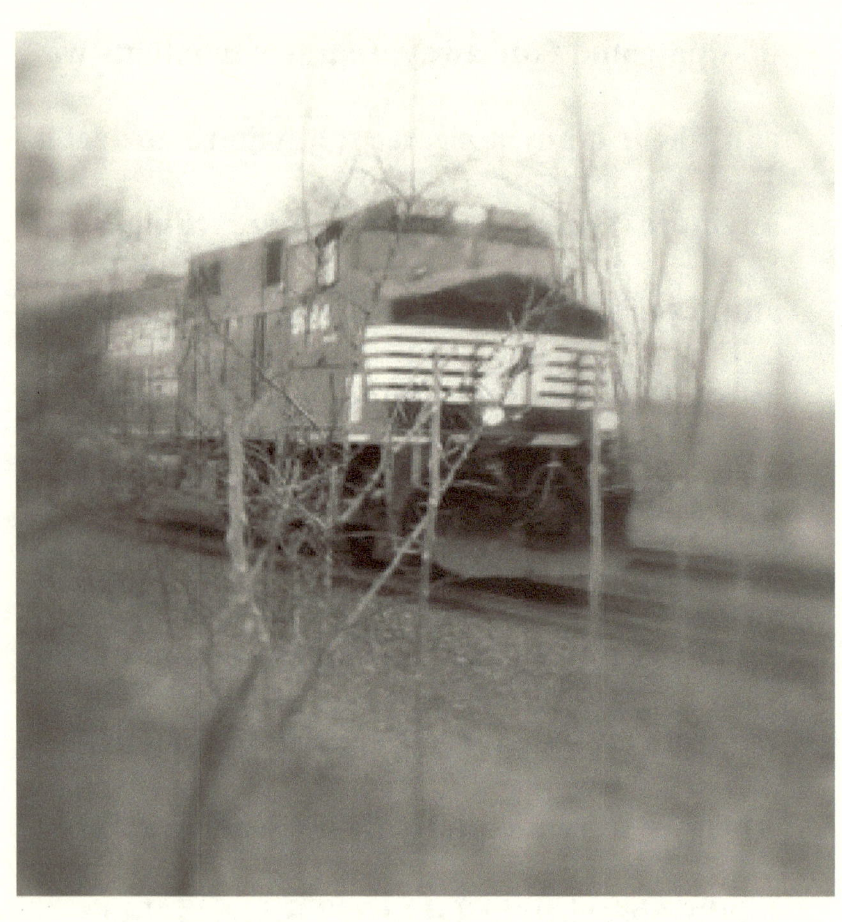

Timeline

Find below an example of a typical beginning meditation session being viewed in a timeline approach. Given a full three minute window of time; our meditation may only last a total of 20 or 30 seconds. Notice that the majority of time we are attempting to experience meditation, we are unfocused and going thru the motions. Then, we have this sense that we are able to absorb all the distractions and a beautiful sense of stillness and enraptured single pointed focus occurs. This experience is meditation.

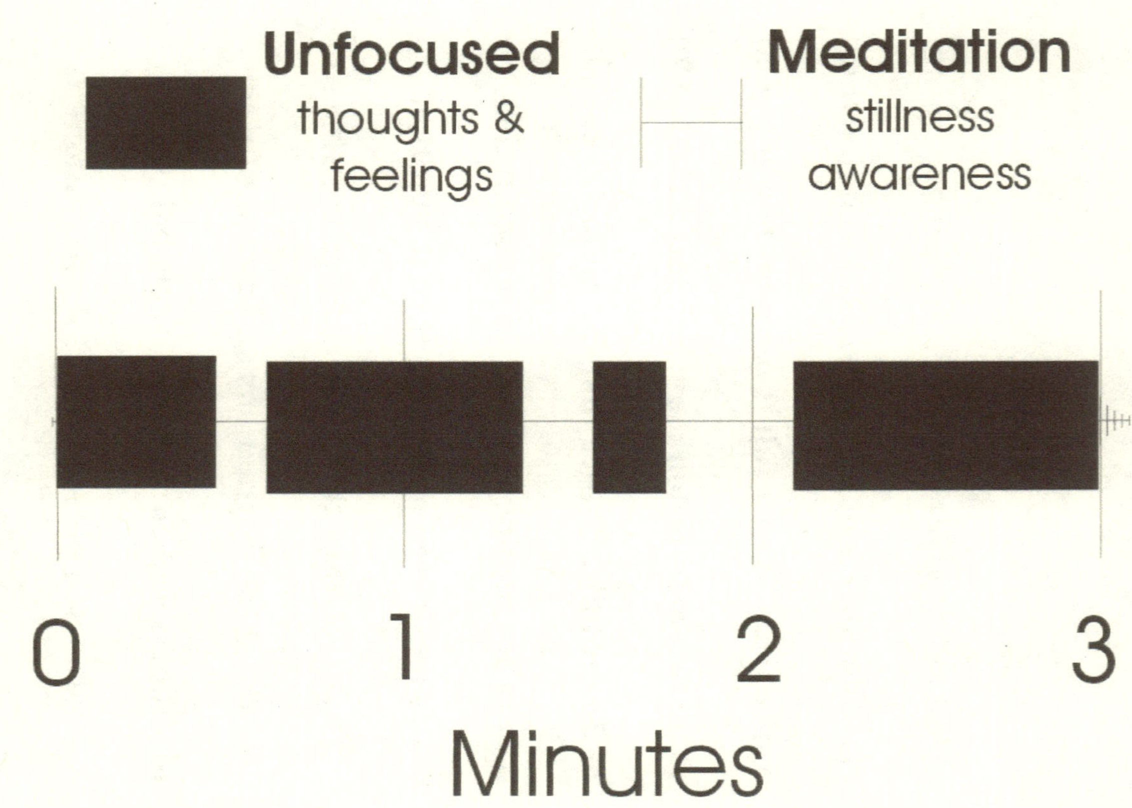

Unfocused
thoughts & feelings
Meditation
stillness awareness
0
1
2
3
Minutes

The thick line represents the period when our conscious mind is active and distracted from our intended purpose, and the small gap represents the times when we are experiencing meditation. Over time those small gaps become larger as our "training" progresses. Only rarely and at a more advanced level of meditation will we experience total one pointed focus for an extended 3 minute period, although it is completely possible and within our reach.

The Pond

I'd like to give another analogy in reference to the active mind, active emotions and active senses as they relate to meditation.

Picture the surface of a pond or lake and we notice that at the surface, the water is still; to the eye it appears to be not moving. The mind is like that during meditation. However, we also know that below the surface of the water there are all kinds of activity going on. Fish are eating, swimming, procreating, giving birth, playing and communicating. Other aquatic life forms are interacting and providing stimulation to the waters underneath the surface, yet the

surface remains still. This stillness is meditation. For us, as our mind is still, all kinds of emotions, mental and physical interactions are occurring at the same time we are experiencing the stillness of meditation. Once the surface of the pond or lake is rippled from a raindrop or a fish splash, the stillness of the surface is disrupted momentarily; the same with our meditation, it is disrupted momentarily. Soon, the surface of the pond or lake stabilizes just like our meditation stabilizes once again.

Remember the timeline? Let's look at another one in relation to the pond or lake.

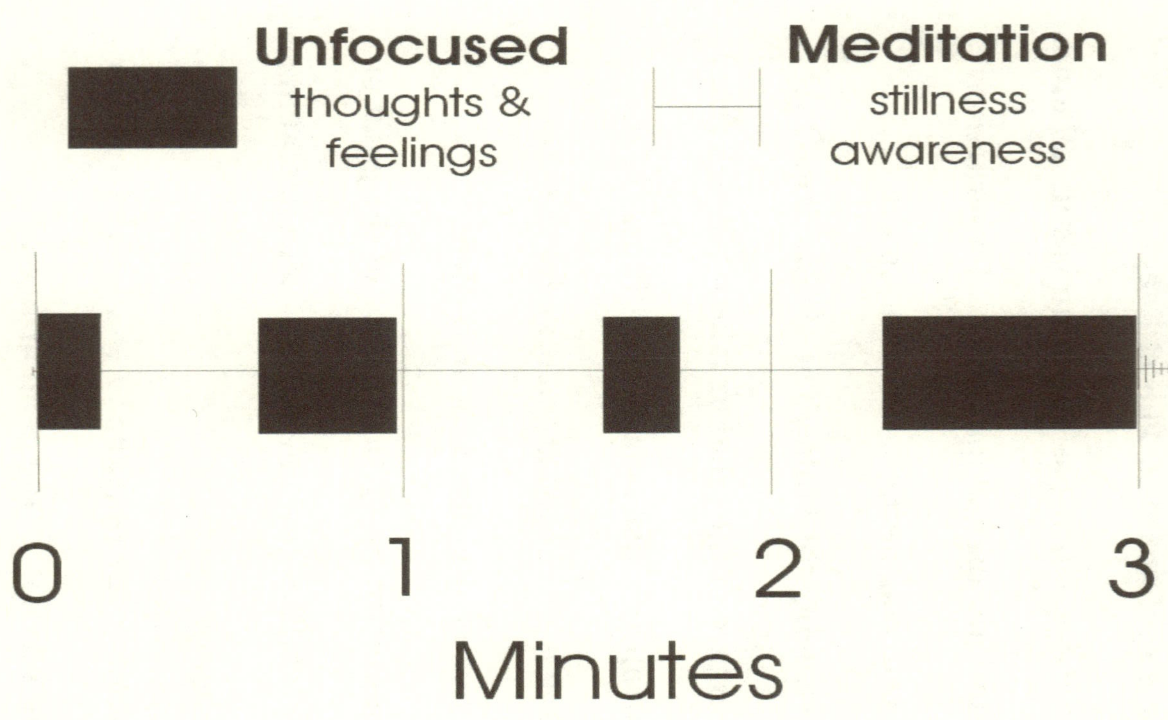
Unfocused
thoughts &
feelings
Meditation
stillness
awareness
0
1
2
3
Minutes

The thick line represents the rippling of the surface of the pond or lake by a raindrop, wind or fish. The gaps represent the time when the surface is still, even though there may be plenty of activity occurring below the surface. During meditation, there is plenty going on below the surface. For one, our active and chatty mind is still going but takes second place to the stillness of meditation. The sensations we experience and our perception of safety take second place to the stillness of meditation; the great thing being, if we sense danger or a safety issue during meditation, our response mechanism automatically kicks in so that we may react properly.

We often wonder just what is the purpose of meditation, why do it at all? Meditation is a natural, innate and normal human function, so we really don't have to wonder why to do it. We just do it.

Most of us have daydreamed. During a daydream we are very caught up in that inner vision and mind experience. The world is going on around us but we are pretty much ignoring all other sensual stimuli during the daydream and becoming the character in the daydream. Daydreaming is very much like meditation and like everything else is OK in moderation. We have all prayed to some extent, we have offered our deepest desires out to a power greater than

ourselves for some measure of fulfillment. While we are praying we are pretty much ignoring all other sensual stimuli and becoming involved as a communicator or feel there is a listener; sometimes having complete expectation of prayer fulfillment and at other times just putting our plea out and hoping for the best result. Prayer and meditation are very similar; however, meditation is less purpose specific. Meditation is done to allow our talents, oftentimes suppressed to take a foothold in our everyday functioning. When the chattering mind plays second fiddle, the orchestra of our extraordinary talents is given center stage, our perceptions are heightened, and our mind

becomes sharp and our emotions clear. This new internal leadership enables us to stay on task, to help us know when to take a rest, when to eat, when and what kind of exercise to do, when to express ourselves and how best to express ourselves, and yes, when to stay silent.

Guided Images

Let's try a sample of some guided images. Read these one at a time, do them until they are indelibly etched into your memory and then do the next step.

Step 1 – While lying in a bed or on the couch or floor, close your eyes and focus on your breath. When I say focus on your breath, I mean listen to it and feel it. Know what your inhale feels like and sounds like. For the sake of this practice, inhale thru the nose and exhale thru the mouth. Know what your exhale feels like and sounds like. During this practice leave a slight gap between your upper and lower lip and leave a slight gap between your upper and

lower teeth. Place the front of your tongue in the back of your lower teeth. Close the mouth thus forcing the inhale thru the nose. As you exhale, lower the bottom jaw slightly, allowing the air out of the body thru the open lips.

A few words about the breath and body: The body is a factory constantly growing new cells, new hair, new fingernails, and toenails, new bones and new skin. The body is basically a big production facility. The inhale is a source of fuel and a natural resource for cell production. Like any other factory, there are toxins and wastes produced as a result of the new cells, skin, bones, etc. These toxins and waste leave the body thru the breath as well as other ways.

Therefore, we do not want to recycle the breath. Let the exhale leave thru the Mouth! We can use this concept on our negative thoughts, negative emotions and negative feelings. Give them all a breath ride on the next exhale out!

Step 2 - Now that we are focusing on our breath, (Note: focus on our breath means listen to and feel the breath) on your next inhale lift the navel upward and during your next exhale let the navel drop naturally. During the next inhale pull the navel downwards towards the spine. On your next exhale, let the navel rise naturally. Repeat this cycle over and over. After a few moments your breath will get quiet and your navel movement will become so slight that

you will hardly be aware of your breath at all. At this point we are in the meditative state. As we go deeper we begin to feel a sensation on the inside of our forehead. During this period we will go into and out of sense awareness. This state is the meditative state. When you come back to physical awareness try to notice all possible sounds about you all at one time. Everything! During this effort we go into the meditative state.

Step 3 - Come to a seated position on the floor or a chair. One way to tell whether your posture is good for a seated meditation is to imagine that you are sitting on a three-prong electrical outlet with the tailbone plugged into

the middle and the two sitting bones plugged into the slots. (This sitting position is attributed to Erich Schiffmann in his book <u>The Spirit and Practice of Moving into Stillness).</u> Nestle yourself into this position with the legs gently crossed. The fingernail of the index finger can gently press against the inside bone of the thumb. Place the rest of the hand palm down on the knees. You will notice that they just kind of fit right. As you are sitting, it is OK to keep adjusting your sitting position from time to time, to keep plugged in, so to speak. Now, visualize in your mind's eye a paper cup dispenser. Picture it over your head. Again, using your constructive imagination, picture a

pointed paper cup from the dispenser drop thru your body to the base of your spine, close to the floor. Fill it with a red color (like the color of an apple for example) until it overflows. Next, picture another pointed cup drop to within a few inches of the red color in the area of the sacrum. Fill it with an orange color until it overflows. Next, visualize another pointed cup drop into the area just below the rib cage and have it fill up with a sun color until it overflows. Next picture another pointed cup drop into an area between the ribs and have it fill up with your own shade of green until it overflows. Now picture one of those pointed cups drop to the area of the throat and let it fill up with your

own shade of blue. Now visualize a pointed paper cup drop to the area of the forehead and let it fill with the color indigo, which is a hue between blue and purple. Finally we picture a pointed paper cup touch the one at the forehead until the top of the cup is level with the top of the head and filling with the color purple.

We can go one step further, but please keep in mind that we may have to do this meditation a few times over the course of a week to deepen the effect and to better visualize the cups and the colors. Our next step in this meditation is to string all the cups together and feel them gently rotating slowly thru the body and spinal area. During this process we will be

experiencing meditation; again, at this stage, possibly for only minutes at a time. We naturally awaken out of this state when necessary or when we are ready.

What color was most prominent or easiest to develop in your mind's eye? Remember that color for later.

How can meditation occur with so much going on in our heads and hearts all the time? How is it possible to stay focused?

May I draw on the concept of loneliness to shed some light? Every one of us has experienced loneliness from time to time. Yet we wonder, how can we be lonely when there is always so much going on around us; if not a

plentiful amount of people, then all the animals, insects, plants, clouds, dewdrops - clearly the list goes on and on. Yet, we experience loneliness with all the possibilities of connection. Meditation has much the same reality. We experience the stillness and focus of meditation while the world goes on around us. Once meditation is truly experienced even loneliness will fade into the past. During meditation, powers and abilities that normally stay dormant are floodgated into an active part of our personality. Ability to perceive the truth is increased, and inner radiant smiles are felt. Although all of life's turmoils are not squelched, the difference between where we would like to

be and the awareness of where we really are is diminished.

Again I would like to stress the concepts of everything in moderation. Meditation included. A three (3) minute meditation once or twice a day is sufficient. We consistently find time to be short and we continually find plenty that needs to be done.

Meditation seems to come easier after a little physical workout. We recommend the Five Tibetans, a fitness ritual of 5 postures repeated up to 21 times each.

These postures combine body and breath awareness, and clean the internal organs the same way that a shower or a bath cleans the

outside of the body. The Five Tibetans can become an excellent 15 minute a day workout.

Full descriptions of the Five Tibetans, along with illustrations are given towards the end of this book.

Now, we can take our meditation to the next level by adding a word to our thought process while we are lying down or in a seated position for meditation. Use the following example whenever you wish. When inhaling, make sure the mouth is closed and the front of the tongue is touching the back of the lower teeth. Silently say the word "HA" as you inhale. Then, as you exhale, drop the lower jaw slightly and whisper the word "THA". Continuously repeat these

words over and over. "HA" on the inhale and "THA" on the exhale. When the mind wanders away, just go back to one of the words until you are focused again. Remember, every time we exhale we get rid of physical and mental toxins, so as we focus more, we become more efficient at getting rid of these toxins. Soon we notice a quietness of the body, breath and mind that becomes meditation, and before we know it, 3 minutes will pass and our meditation experience is complete.

Another word to use is the Sanskrit (an ancient Indian Language) word for the color that you were able to create most – the one you liked the best of the seven. These are listed here.

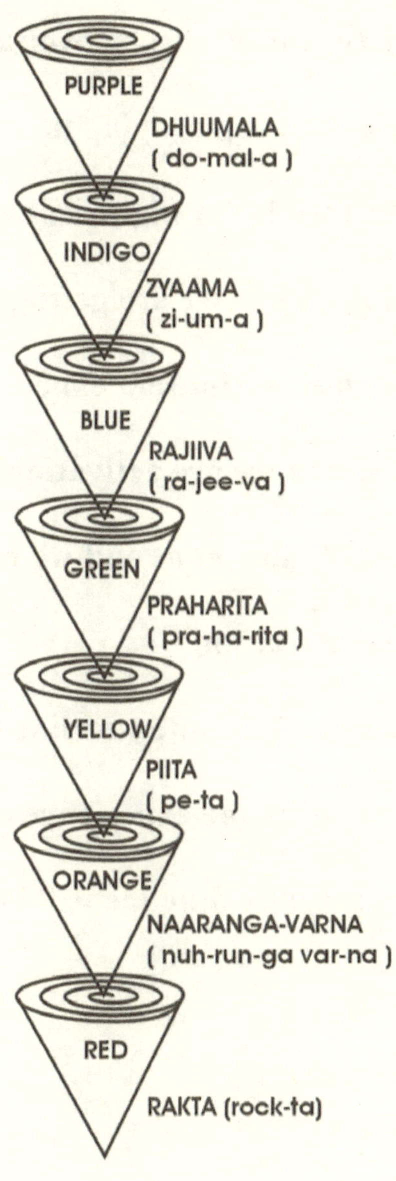
PURPLE
DHUUMALA
(do-mal-a)
INDIGO
ZYAAMA
(zi-um-a)
BLUE
RAJIIVA
(ra-jee-va)
GREEN
PRAHARITA
(pra-ha-rita)
YELLOW
PIITA
(pe-ta)
ORANGE
NAARANGA-VARNA
(nuh-run-ga var-na)
RED
RAKTA (rock-ta)

Chose your favorite word or color and continuously repeat that word over and over again as you are sitting or lying in a meditative position. When we feel a slight sensation behind the forehead we know we are getting somewhere in our meditation experience. During meditation we are activating brain cells that are normally dormant and we become aware of that activation.

Remember the 3 minute timeline from before? As we enjoy the experience of meditation more, our timeline will begin to look like this:

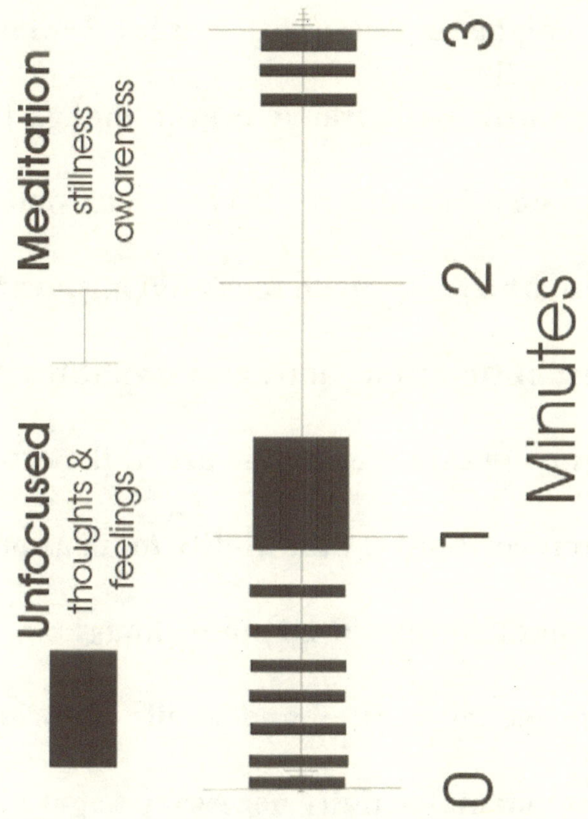

In the above illustration, the black lines represent periods of distraction and the open areas represent time of single pointed focus and deep meditation.

Imagine the possibility of a full 3 minutes of focus with no distractions even though they may go on all around us. If you ever wondered how an athlete is able to focus during a very important time in a game, we inevitably find them saying that they are aware of the external distractions, but that the ability to focus on one thing that drowns out all other thoughts, sounds, feelings, tastes, and smells, allowing the surge of mental activity necessary to get the body to perform to the best of its ability.

We all have moments of great distraction where we can use the principles learned in this book to minimize distractions and thus allow our inner powers to guide us thru the ordinary

travails of our daily life in a way that brings a smile to our face as we go along.

The Smile

While sitting in an easy sitting pose or lying in a comfortable position, allow a smile to come to your face but don't use the lips to express the smile. Get the feel of a smile throughout your face. Now, take that smile feeling further into the body. Let it go thru the neck, across the shoulders, thru the arms and hands. Create that same sensation thru the ribs down to the hips, thru the legs into the feet. Inhale and allow your whole body to feel like a smile. Now let the lips curve up to complete a full body smile.

The Five Tibetans

Begin this fitness ritual at a slow pace. Do seven repetitions a day for one month. Do 14 repetitions a day during the second month, and the do 21 repetitions starting after two months. Spend no more than 15 minutes a day on the exercise ritual regardless of whether you are a beginner or an advanced practitioner.

Approach it as fun and not as a chore.

Give yourself some time of improve. Most importantly; inhale or exhale with each movement. Generally we inhale for strength and exhale for flexibility. For the purpose of this fitness ritual; inhale thru your nose and

exhale thru your unrestrained mouth whenever possible.

First Tibetan- Twirling

Remember when you were a child and you would spin around in a circle when playing outdoors in the yard or park? NASA astronauts go thru a spinning exercise to improve their ability to maintain their balance.

The Posture----- Stand with your feet about shoulder width apart. Place your arms out to the sides like airplane wings. Turn your right palm to face the floor and your left palm to face the ceiling. Keep your eyes focused on the fingernails of the right hand. Do not move the eyes. Inhale and turn slowly counterclockwise

making a complete circle. Exhale. For the first month repeat this posture 7 times.

When finished twirling, allow your right arm to rest across the front of your body and let the left arm to rest across the lower back. Look down at your left foot until you feel completely stable. Bring your feet back together, hands together in prayer position. Inhale thru your nose as you bring your hands up toward the ceiling. Exhale thru the mouth as you bring your arms down and back into prayer position. Do this champion breath a total of three times. This completes Posture 1.

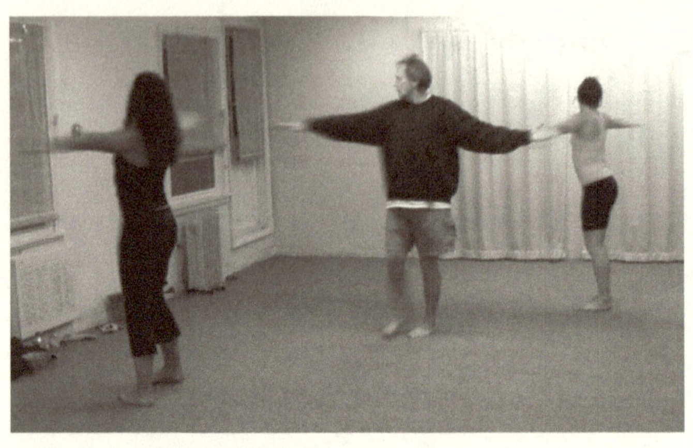

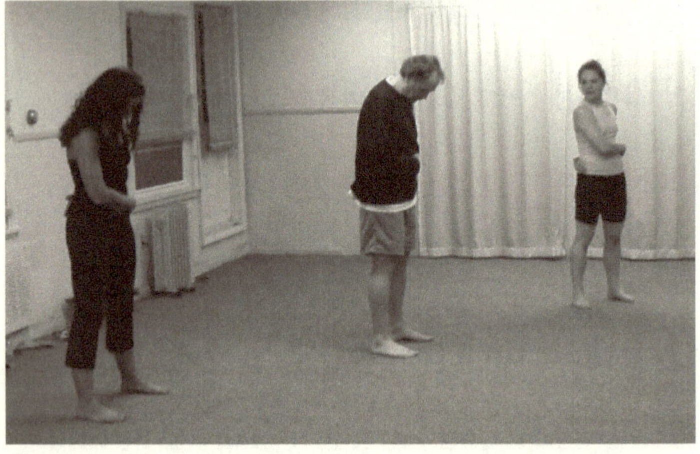

For the second month repeat this posture 14 times. After the second month repeat this posture 21 times.

Modification for the beginner:

Spinal twist – Stand with your feet about shoulder width apart. Place your arms out to the sides loosely like airplane wings. Instead of twirling in a circle; simply swing the arms from side to side letting the heels lift and the knees bend for comfort.

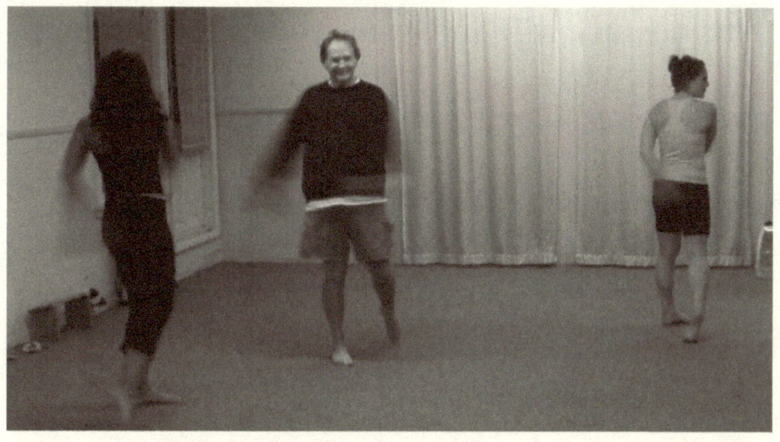

Listen to and feel your breath. For the first month repeat this posture 7 times.

Bring your feet back together, hands together in prayer position. Inhale thru your nose as you bring your hands up toward the ceiling. Exhale thru the mouth as you bring your arms down and back into prayer position. Do this champion breath a total of three times.

This completes Posture 1.

This posture will limber up your spine and get good energy flowing thru your body. For the second month repeat this posture 14 times. After the second month repeat this posture 21 times.

Second Tibetan- Core Lift

Lie on your back with legs straight. Place your hands beside your hips or just slightly under them with the palms facing down; fingers pointing toward the feet. During the inhale; simply lift the navel. As you exhale thru the mouth; lift the legs straight up to a 90 degree angle. In addition; lift the head off the floor - chin in towards the chest. Leave the shoulders on the floor! For the first month repeat this posture 7 times.

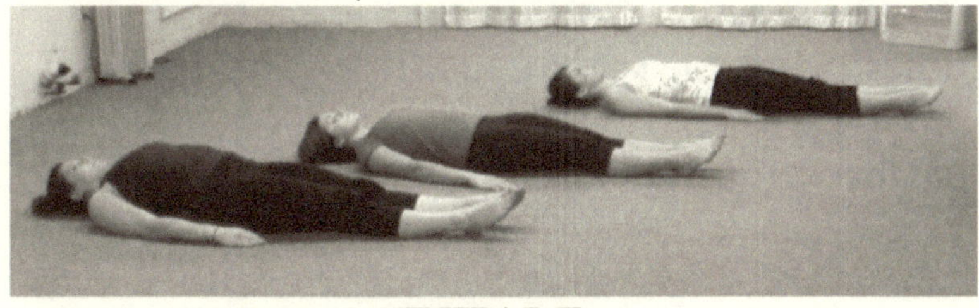

INHALE

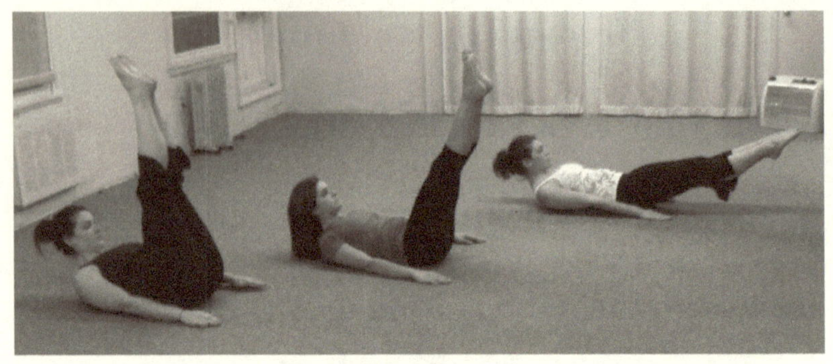

EXHALE

When finished, lie flat on your back and bring your hands up toward the sky; touch the tips of the thumbs and fingers together and place the hands over the navel. Take three breaths.

This completes posture two.

For the second month repeat this posture 14 times. After the second month repeat this posture 21 times.

Modification for the beginner:

Lie on your back with the knees bent and feet flat on the floor. During the inhale; simply lift the navel. As you exhale thru the mouth; lift the bent legs up off the floor. In addition; lift the head off the floor - chin in towards the chest. Leave the shoulders on the floor! For the first month repeat this posture 7 times.

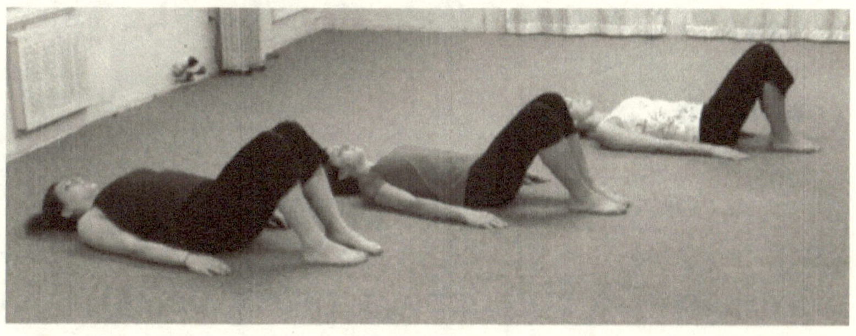

INHALE

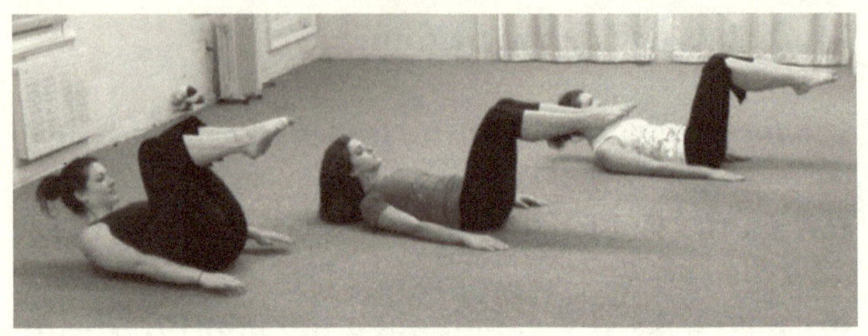

EXHALE

When finished, lie flat on your back and bring your hands up toward the sky; touch the tips of the thumbs and fingers together and place the hands over the navel. Take three breaths. This completes Posture two.

This posture will increase core strength and release tension held in the neck and shoulders. For the second month repeat this posture 14 times. After the second month repeat this posture 21 times.

Third Tibetan – Backbend

Kneel on your towel or folded mat with your knees about eight inches apart, Support your lower back by placing your hands on the sides of your lower back with thumbs pointed out and fingers straight down. Keep them there. As you inhale thru the nose drop you head backwards and lift the chest up towards the ceiling. As you exhale; slowly bring the chin back in to touch the chest. For the first month repeat this posture 7 times.

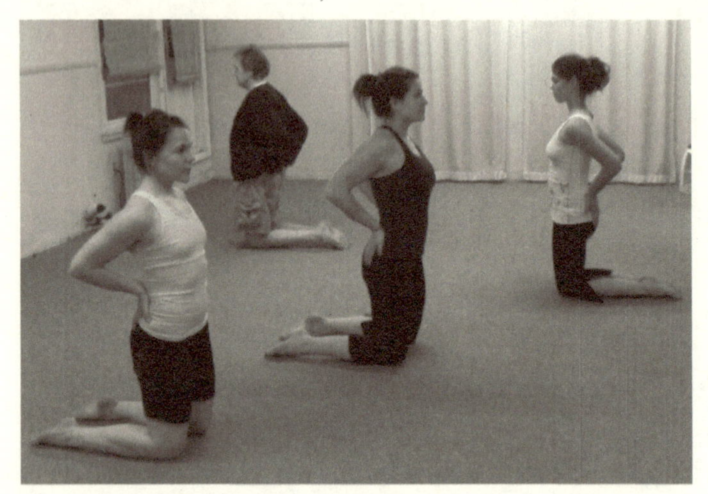

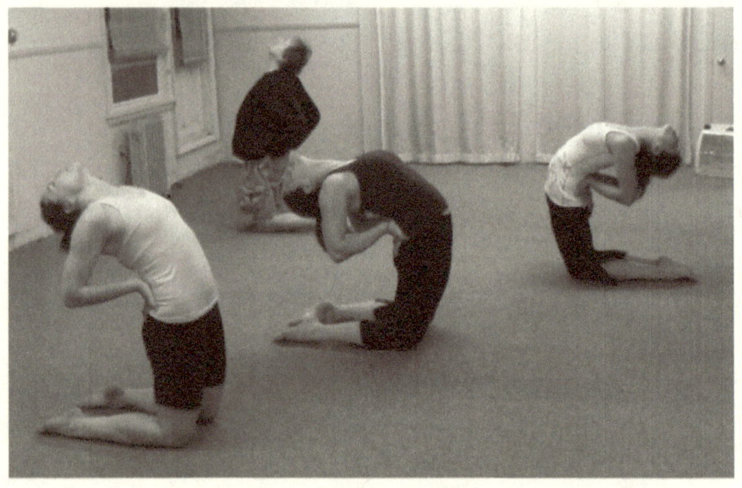

INHALE

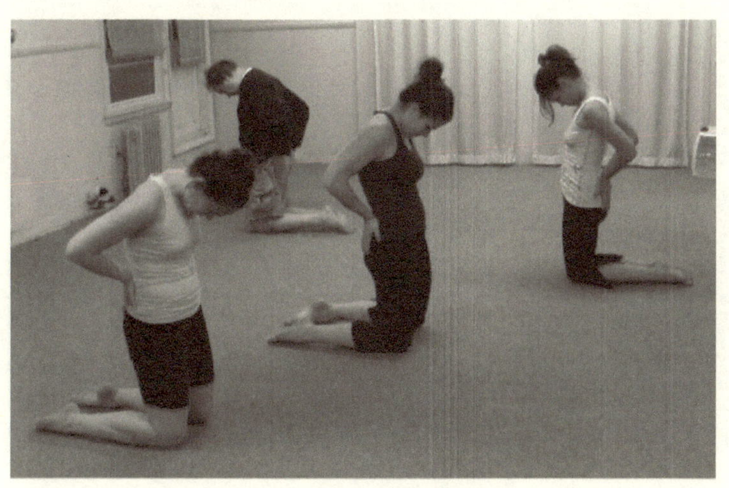

EXHALE

When finished; sit on your heels or comfortably on the floor. Dig the sides of your hands (palms up) into the hip bones and lean your torso forward with your forehead reaching toward the floor. Take three breaths.

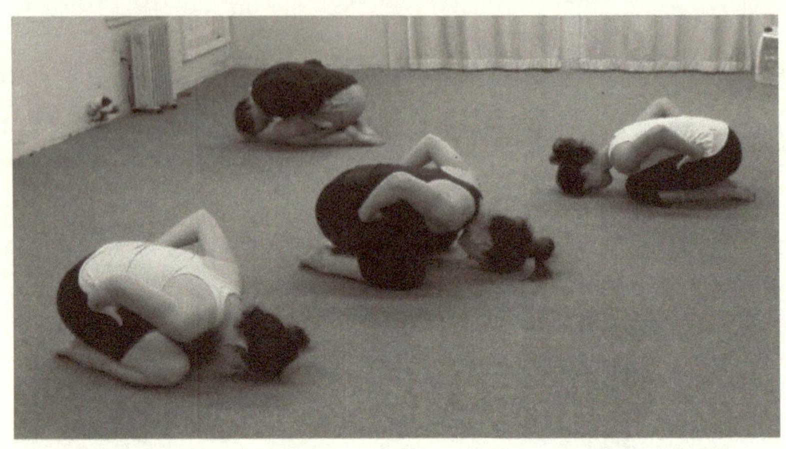

This completes posture 3.

Twenty four hours a day; seven days a week we forward bend. This posture takes the spine in the opposite direction and has an effect similar to what I call Nature's Prozac; i.e. Nature's anti-depressant. For the second month repeat this posture 14 times. After the second month repeat this posture 21 times.

<u>Posture three is the same for beginner and advanced.</u>

Fourth Tibetan – Table

Sit on the floor with your back straight and your legs out in front of you with your feet about shoulder width apart. Place your hands on the floor directly beside your hips; palms down; fingers pointing toward your feet. As you inhale thru your nose lift your hips up toward the ceiling; the hands stay on the floor; arms perpendicular to the floor, supporting the torso. Exhale thru the mouth and bring the hips down to the floor directly beside the hands. Bring the chin gently into the chest. For the first month repeat this posture 7 times.

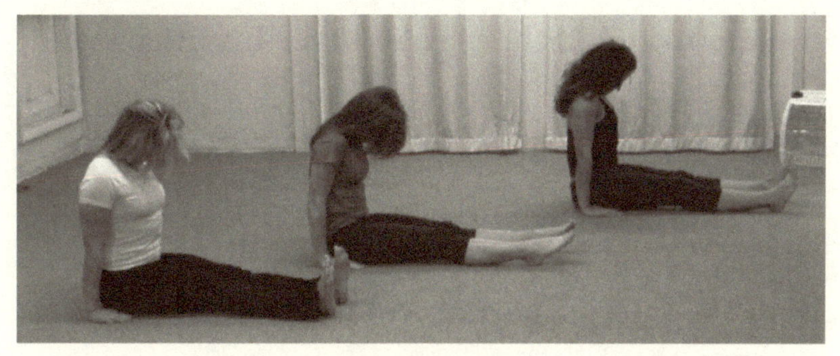

EXHALE

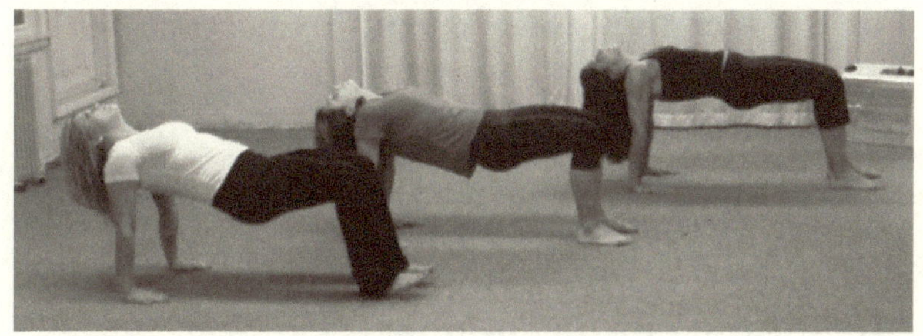

INHALE

When finished lie back on the floor, bend your knees and have the bottom of the feet touch each other. Place the arms over the head on the floor and touch the tips of the thumbs and

fingers to each other. Take three breaths, eyes open or closed.

This completes posture four. This posture will firm the triceps, getting rid of the jiggles and firm the gludial muscles.

For the second month repeat this posture 14 times. After the second month repeat this posture 21 times.

<u>Modification for the beginner:</u>

Lie on the floor with your knees bent upward, feet flat on the floor. Place the arms on the floor beside the hips with the palms facing downward; fingers pointing toward the feet.

As you inhale bring the hips up as high as is comfortable. As you exhale thru the mouth

bring the hips slowly back to the floor one vertebrae at a time. Repeat seven times.

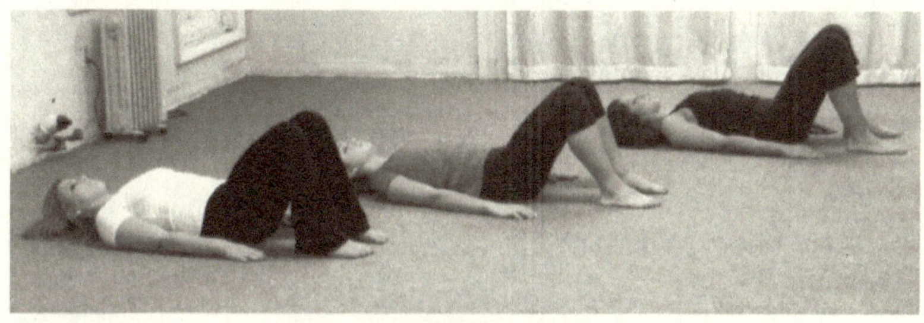

EXHALE

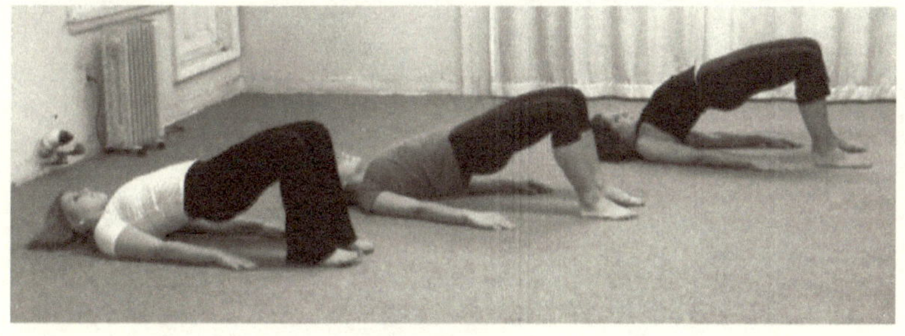

INHALE

When finished lie back on the floor, bend your knees; have the bottom of the feet touch each other. Place the arms over the head on the floor

and touch the tips of the thumbs and fingers to each other. Take three breaths, eyes open or closed. This completes posture four.

This posture will firm the gludial muscles.

For the second month repeat this posture 14 times. After the second month repeat this posture 21 times.

Fifth Tibetan – Spine Strengthening

Start on all fours; hands and knees. Have the hands shoulder width apart; nice distance between the thumb and little finger without pressure or strain. Have the feet about shoulder width apart. Now left your knees off the floor and straighten your legs. If you feel stiff; bend your right knee to stretch your left leg and then vice versa. Distribute your weight equally forward and back; don't put all the weight on your wrists; lets the fingers take some of the weight. As you inhale thru your nose; bring your hips down toward the floor and lift your head up toward the ceiling. Arms remain straight. As you exhale thru the mouth; bring

the hips up toward the ceiling; bring the heels down toward the floor and bring the chin gently in toward the chest. Arms stay straight, supporting the torso. For the first month repeat this posture seven times.

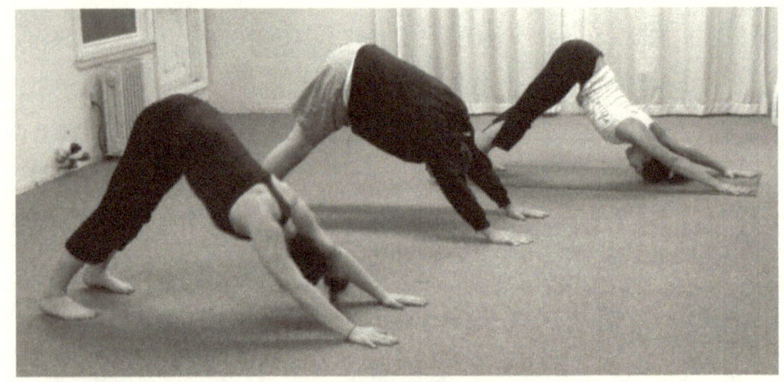

EXHALE

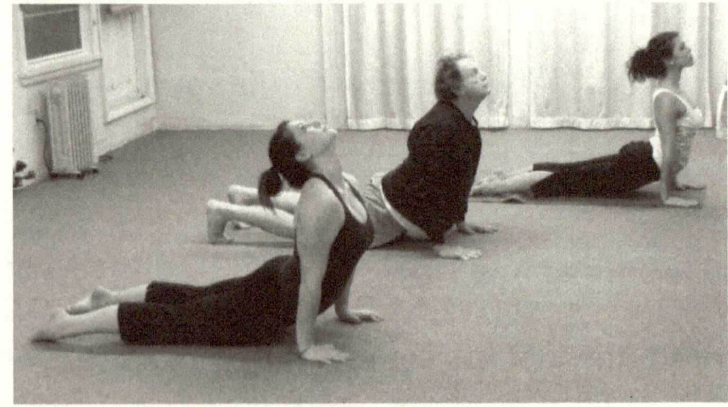

INHALE

Now, come to a standing position. Turn toward the East and lift the hands (palms up) toward the ceiling. Turn towards the South. Lower the hands back down toward the floor turning the palms down. Lift the hands (palms up) toward the ceiling. Turn toward the West. Lower the hands back down toward the floor turning the palms down. Lift the hands (palms up) toward the ceiling. Turn towards the North. Lower the hands back down toward the floor turning the palms down. Lift the hands (palms up) toward the ceiling. Turn towards the East. Lower the hands back down toward the floor turning the palms down. This posture will strengthen the spine and improve your overall posture.

This completes the five Tibetans.

For the second month repeat this posture 14 times. After the second month repeat this posture 21 times.

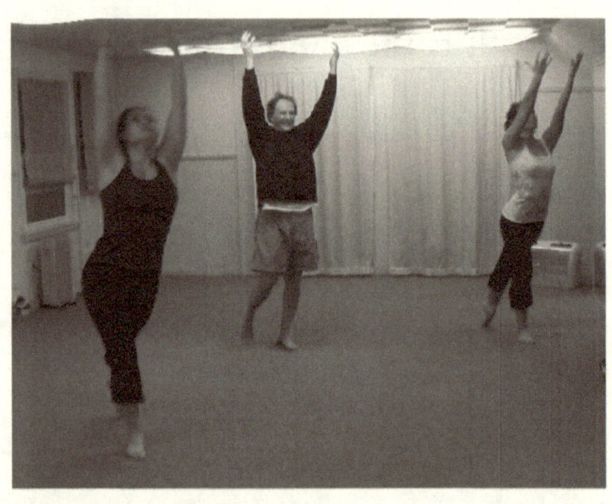

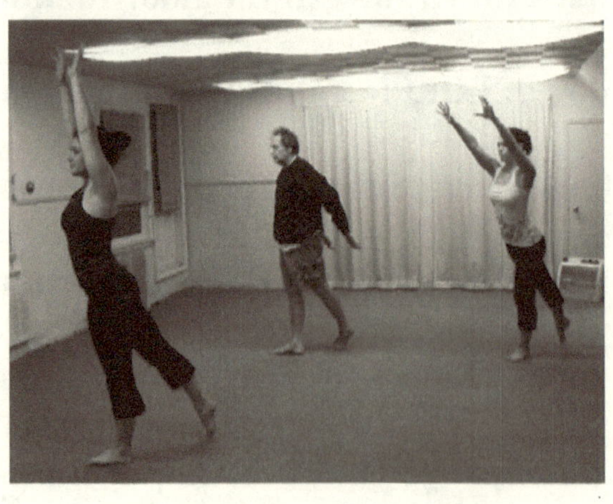

Modification for the beginner:

Sit on your heels letting your hips rest on your heels with your arms stretched forward palms facing down. As you inhale thru the nose move forward thru your arms until you lift your torso off the floor and the arms go perpendicular to the floor supporting the torso. As you exhale thru the mouth; return to the original position with the hips resting on the heels. Repeat this posture seven times during the first month.

Come to a standing position. Turn toward the East and lift the hands (palms up) toward the ceiling. Turn towards the South. Lower the hands back down toward the floor turning the palms down. Lift the hands (palms up) toward

the ceiling. Turn toward the West. Lower the hands back down toward the floor turning the palms down. Lift the hands (palms up) toward the ceiling. Turn towards the North. Lower the hands back down toward the floor turning the palms down. Lift the hands (palms up) toward the ceiling. Turn towards the East. Lower the hands back down toward the floor turning the palms down.

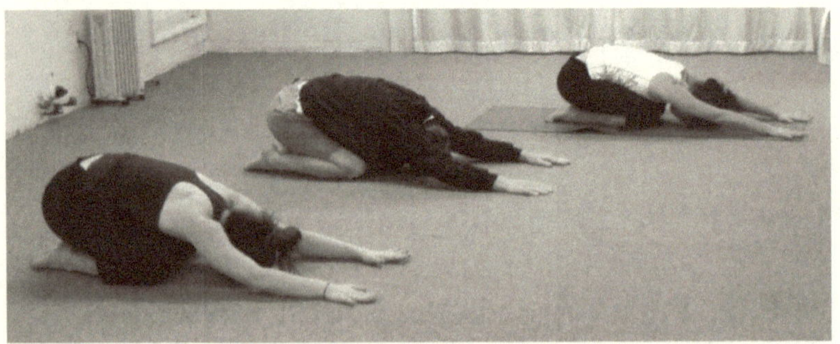

EXHALE

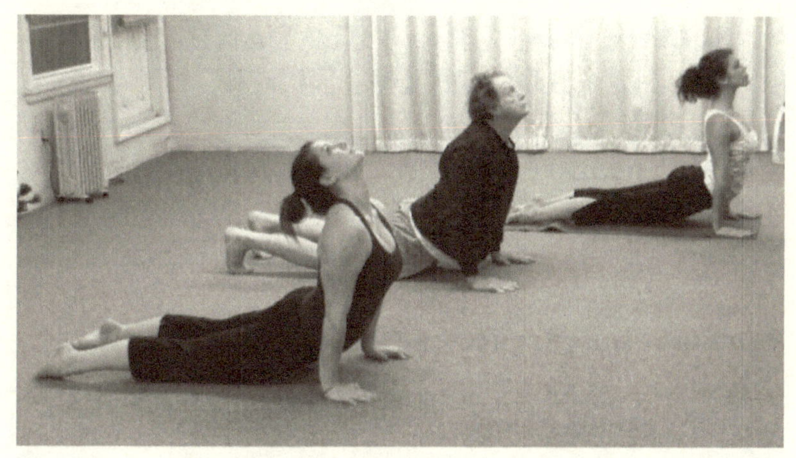

INHALE

This completes the five Tibetans.

This posture will strengthen the spine and improve your overall posture.

For the second month repeat this posture 14 times. After the second month repeat this posture 21 times.

BONUS POSTURE- TULADANDASANA BALANCING STICK

Use this posture when you have only a few minutes a day to devote to exercise. It is an excellent posture for the heart and cardiovascular system.

In a standing position; feet together nicely; bring your arms up over your head and interlace your fingers with the index fingers pointed up toward the ceiling. Step forward with your right foot about tow feet. Plant he right foot on the floor and come up on the toes of the left foot. Straighten the body; keep the standing leg straight; bring the torso down and the back leg up equal amounts.

If possible bring the leg and torso parallel to the floor and stretch your arms forward and leg back strongly for 10 seconds. Be straight like a stick. If you should begin to lose your balance simply bring the arms up and leg down until you feel confident and balanced and stretch from there for 10 seconds.

Come back to the original position with the arms up over the head; feet together nicely and repeat the posture on the other side. This posture has the ability to raise the Heart rate about 20 beats per minute and improve your circulation. Try it and see!

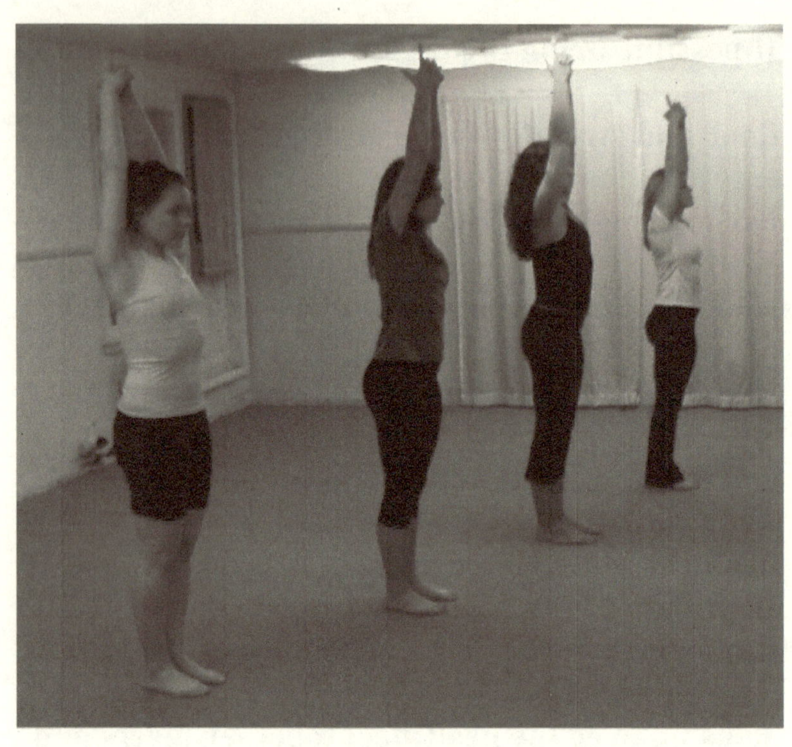

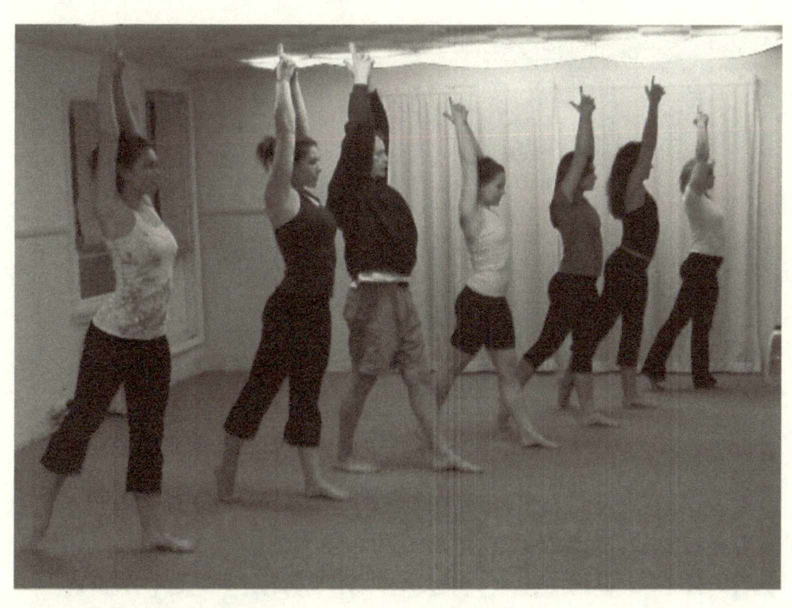

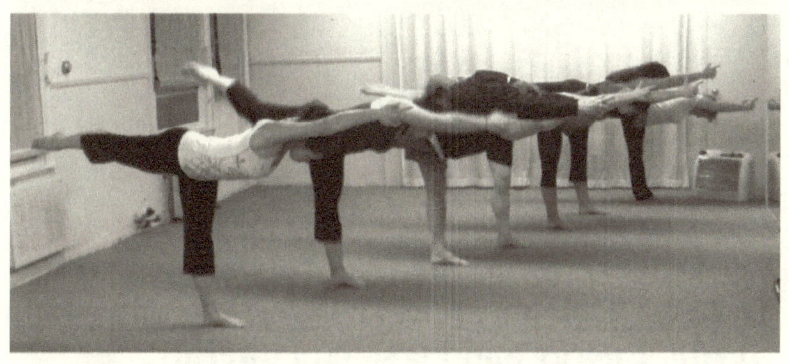

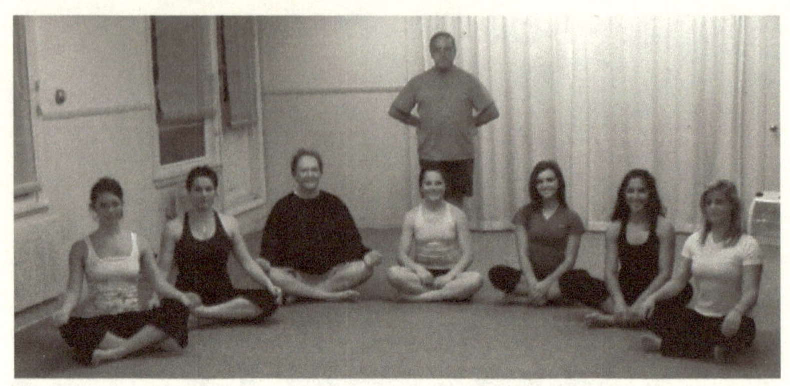

Pictured from Left to Right: Taylor Rees, Rebecca Rockey, Randy Earhart, Lauren Coughlin, Chelsey Pagana, Kacie Heilman, Elizabeth Praedin. Standing: Doug Hayward

Reference book for the Five Tibetans is: The Five Tibetans: Five Dynamic Exercises for Health, Energy and Personal Power by Christopher S. Kilham; or The Ancient Secret of the Fountain of Youth: Book 1 by Peter Kelder and Bernie S. Siegel

www.ingramcontent.com/pod-product-compliance
Lightning Source LLC
LaVergne TN
LVHW050941080826
845145LV00004B/1365

* 9 7 8 0 9 7 2 1 1 1 6 2 1 *